MEDITERRENEAN DIET

As you can tell, Mediterranean foods differ depending on which country you're in. Nevertheless, these foods are known worldwide and people will travel from near and far just to indulge in their goodness.

Table of Contents

LUNCH

Rice, Couscous Salad or Pasta

Rice, pasta and couscous are both low potassium alternatives to potato and make a filling alternative to bread. Try cold cooked rice, pasta or couscous mixed with tuna, ham or chicken and a range of vegetables such as sweet corn, cucumber, olives, peppers and some mayo. You could try flavoring it with some herbs or spices, for example dried basil, parsley, paprika or even curry powder. A dash of salad dressing, spoonful of pesto or stirring in soft white cream cheese can give it extra flavour.

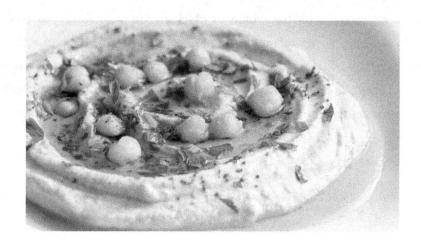

Oatcake or Rice Toppings

It is possible to use oat and rice cakes as a good snack and here are some suggestions for healthy toppings that are also small in potassium and phosphate.

Ingredients:

Cottage cheese mixed with pineapple (canned and drained) or mixed with sweet corn (canned)

- Cottage cheese mixed with chicken, peas (pre-boiled or canned) and thyme

- Cream cheese mixed with garlic and chive or parsley or any other herb or spice

- Lean ham with cream cheese

- Egg mayonnaise

- Tuna mayonnaise

- Tinned fish (without bones as this makes them high in phosphate)

Healthy Porridge

If you're interested in weight loss, this porridge can be a nice option because it's small in calories and high in fiber that will assist you feel full longer, so you're less likely to snack before dinner. If you are on phosphate restraint, you may want to attempt soy or rice milk to substitute skimmed milk as it is smaller in phosphate and generally low in fat.

Ingredients:

- 35 g of porridge oats
- 100ml of skimmed milk
- 100ml of water
- 1/2 grated apple

Preparation Technique:

1. 1. After heating the pan, mix all the ingredients in the saucepan and boil 3-4 min.

2. Alternatively boil for about 1-2 minutes in the microwave, stirring at intervals of 30 seconds.

Granola

1. Home-made Granolas: Because of the elevated content of nuts and dried fruit, many shops purchased granolas are inappropriate if you follow potassium and phosphate constraints. Here's a easy step by step method to create your own alternative oat breakfast that can be served with milk, yogurt or stewed fruit.

Here we have added dried cranberries as they are naturally smaller in potassium than other dried fruits but without them they will taste just as nice.

Ingredients to serve up to 10 people:

- 4 tablespoons of sunflower or vegetable oil
- 2 tablespoons of clear honey or golden syrup

- 1 table spoon of lemon juice

- 2 tablespoons of soft brown sugar

- 300 g (10and half oz) rolled oats

Preparation Technique:

1. Oven pre-heat to 140 ° C (120 ° C)/275 ° F

2. Melt the oil, honey / sirup, citrus juice and sugar over low heat in a big saucepan. The goal is not to allow the mixture bubble to melt and mix together the ingredients. Add the oats, then stir well.

3. The mixture should be spread in an even layer on a baking tray (you may need two baking trays depending on their size. For 30-40 minutes, It should be baked in the oven until crisp. Check the granola every 10 minutes and stir to ensure even baking.

4. Once cooked and cooled, add a few handfuls of dried cranberries

Almond Green Goddess Dressing

Ingredients

1 cup of almonds pre-splashed for 8 hours

2 cups cleaned water or light vegetable stock

1/2 pack of parsley, cleaved

2 scallions, hacked

2 cloves garlic

Juice of 2 lemons

Preparation

Tamari (wheat free), Braggs or Dr. Bronner's fluid aminos or ocean salt to taste

Pour 1 cup of water or stock into blender and include lemon juice, parsley, garlic, and flavoring. Mix well. Include 1/4 of the almonds and mix. Gradually include remaining almonds and water and keep mixing until you have a smooth, velvety dressing. Refrigerate before serving.

Sunflower Dressing

Ingredients

1 cup sunflower seeds

1 cup spring water juice of 2 lemons

2 scallions, slashed

1/2 bundle of parsley, slashed

2 Tbs. crisp tarragon or 1/2 tsp. dried thyme

2 cloves garlic

Preparation

Kelp or Braggs 'fluid aminos' to taste

Spot half of the sunflower seeds in blender. Include remaining fixings and mix. Include remaining sunflower seeds while mixing. In the event that dressing is excessively thick, include extra water. Refrigerate before serving.

Dill Tahini Dressing

Ingredients

1 cup tahini, crude

1/3 cup new lemon juice

1/4 cup tamari, Bragg's fluid aminos, or ocean salt to taste

2 Tbs. new minced dill or 1/2 tsp. dried dill

1 Tbs. garlic powder cleansed water or light vegetable stock

Preparation

Blend tahini and lemon squeeze and mix. Include dill, garlic, and flavoring. Mix while including water or stock until wanted smooth consistency is acquired. Refrigerate before serving.

Curried Pumpkin Dip

Ingredients

2 cups ground pumpkin or butternut squash

1/2 avocado, cut

1 little tomato, cleaved

1 celery stalk with leaves, cut

2 scallions, cleaved

2 Tbs. Tamari

BraggsTM fluid aminos, or ocean salt to taste

2 tsp. curry powder

2 Tbs. lemon juice

1/2 cup filtered water

Preparation

Put water in blender and include vegetables. Mix until smooth. Include lemon squeeze and curry powder and season to taste. Include extra water if excessively thick. Refrigerate before serving.

Spinach Dip

Ingredients

1-1/2 cups spinach

1 ready avocado, cut juice of 1 lemon

1/2 cup purged water

1 tsp. dried mustard powder

2 Tbs. crisp basil or 1/2 tsp. dried ocean salt to taste

Preparation

Add water and avocado to blender. Mix until smooth. Include remaining fixings. Modify flavoring to taste.

Refrigerate before serving.

Hank's Pesto Sauce

Ingredients

2 oz. crisp ginger (stripped)

8 enormous cloves garlic

1/2 bundle of parsley

1 cup natural sesame oil (e.g., Spectrum Naturals or Flora brand) ocean salt to taste

Preparation

Include ginger, garlic, and parsley to nourishment processor and slash into fine bits. Marinate the hacked vegetables in the sesame oil for 10-20 minutes and add ocean salt to taste.

Sandwich

Preparation

These days sandwiches could be made up of bread, pitta, wraps, rolls or any other bread range available. The best choice is always wholemeal as it includes more fiber, but if you prefer white then occasionally choose this choice. Here are some proposed fillings that provide excellent protein sources perfect for patients with dialysis:

- Ham and cream cheese

- Chicken pesto and mayonnaise

- Tuna mayo with cucumber

- Coronation chicken (chicken blended with mayonnaise and some curry powder)

- Cheese (within allowance), a tiny quantity of salad and mayonnaise

- Egg and cress

- Sliced beef and horseradish or mustard

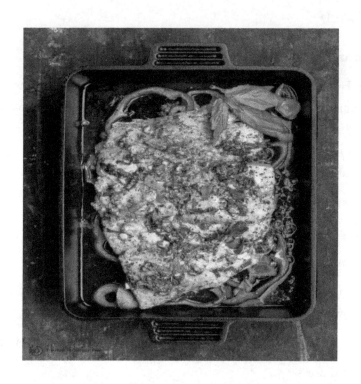

Quiche

Preparation

Because quiche is produced with protein-friendly eggs, then quiche makes a nice dinner to replace the protein lost during dialysis. While ready-made quiches are fine, try a low /reduced salt option (less than 1.5 g per 100 g). You may want to prevent the pastry and boil your own quiche using the' pastry-less quiche recipe' in this book's vegetarian chapter if you are attempting to lose weight. For example, the following foods all contain tiny amounts of chocolate are Small milk bar (wafer or biscuit-based like Taxi, Kitkat or Penguin because they have less than the elevated chocolate of phosphate), Digestive chocolate cookies, Chocolate cereal bar, Chocolate cake, etc.Cookie chocolate chips (prevent double chocolate chips)

Crisp Corn

Preparation

For example, Skips, Dorritos, Monster Munch, Quavers, Wotsits, poppadoms, Tortilla chips (if you try to lose weight, choose low-calorie alternatives such as about 100kcal per packet). Naturally, crisps are high in salt, so restrict how many times you appreciate them.

Baked Lemon Garlic Salmon

Preparation

Perfectly tender, flaky baked salmon with a homemade lemon and garlic sauce. This recipe takes very little prep and less than 20 minutes to cook.

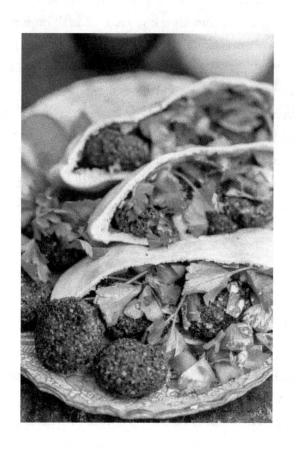

Greek-Style Eggplant Recipe

Preparation

This simple vegan eggplant stew with chickpeas and tomatoes is all the comfort. And you'll love the Greek flavors thanks to a little extra virgin olive oil and a combination of warm spices including oregano, paprika, and a pinch of cinnamon.

Chicken-Shawarma

Preparation

This easy baked chicken Shawarma will transport you to the streets of the Middle East! Loads of flavor. The secret is in the simple homemade Shawarma spice mixture.

Easy Baked Fish with Garlic and Basil

The secret to this juicy fish is in the quick fish marinade with a few spices, garlic, fresh basil, a little citrus and extra virgin olive oil.

Veggie Scramble

1–2 eggs for every individual, mixed with green onions, tomatoes, cleaved bokchoy or other verdant green, and ringer peppers.

Preparation:

1 pear

Bunch (1 oz.) toasted pumpkin seeds.

Lentil soup

It is presented with 2 cups of steamed vegetables (broccoli, kale, carrots, and onions).

Preparation:

Sprinkle olive oil plate of mixed greens dressing on gently steamed vegetables. Or then again 4 oz. cold or hot salmon (or chicken, fish, or tofu), served more than 2–3 cups blended greens, tomatoes, cucumber, carrots, broccoli, or other crisp vegetables.

Lemon Dill vinaigrette.

Preparation:

• Hard-bubbled egg cut and sprinkled with ocean salt and slashed level leaf parsley.

• Red ringer pepper strips, celery or carrot sticks. A bunch of almonds is additionally a nibble choice.

• 4 oz. serving of fish, chicken, turkey or other meat presented with a heated yam or sweet potato and a blended nursery plate of mixed greens. or on the other hand.

• Pasta (produced using buckwheat, rice, amaranth, or quinoa as opposed to wheat) bested with severe greens —, for example, broccoli rabe or arugula—in addition to slashed zucchini, pine nuts or fragmented almonds, garlic, lemon squeeze and pizzazz, salt, and pepper.

• Include a grinding of pecorino Romano or crisp Parmesan, whenever wanted.

• Regular natural products: In summer, attempt nectarines and fruits, or grapes and melon; in winter, attempt broiled pears or prepared apples.

Asparagus ı la Sweet Lemon

PER SERVING: 128.4

Lemon is a great flavor to add to most dishes, and the nutmeg adds a surprising sweetness to the asparagus.

Serves 4

Substitutions

You could attempt this formula with green beans.

Ingredients

2 bunches asparagus (about 1 pound)

Juice of 1 medium lemon

3 tablespoons olive oil

½ teaspoon sea salt

¼ teaspoon black pepper

¼ teaspoon ground nutmeg

1 tablespoon ground cashews (for garnish)

Preparation

Wash the asparagus, cut off the ends, and steam until the stems are cooked but still a little firm.

Mix together in a bowl lemon juice, oil, sea salt, pepper, and nutmeg.

Arrange the asparagus on a serving dish and drizzle with the lemon juice mixture.

Baba Ghanoush

Baba ghanoush it is extraordinary for plunging and as a side to any meat dish.

Ingredients

1 enormous eggplant or 2 little eggplants

¼ cup in addition to 1 storing tablespoon tahini (sesame seed spread)

½–1 teaspoon salt

1–2 garlic cloves, minced

2 tablespoons crisp lemon juice

1/8 teaspoon ground cumin

¼ teaspoon dark pepper

Paprika for decorate

Parsley for embellish

Preparation

Preheat the stove to 350 F. Leaving the eggplant entirety, prepare it on a heating sheet until delicate, around 30 minutes. (For a smoother baba ghanoush, expel the strip from the eggplant before mixing.)

Permit to cool to room temperature.

Cut eggplant(s) open, evacuate the same number of seeds as you can, and cut the remaining substance into 3D squares. Mix all fixings in blender until smooth.

Topping with parsley and paprika, and present with rice wafers, non-wheat bread, or plunging vegetables, for example, carrots and celery.

Serves 6

Basil Pesto

This adaptable pesto can be utilized on rice saltines, on non-wheat pasta, in egg dishes, in servings of mixed greens, or with whatever else your taste buds can cook up.

Spread it on a spelt pizza outside layer, or substitute it in any dish that requires a tomato-based marinara sauce. You can twofold or triple the formula and solidify the pesto in containers for some time later.

Ingredients

4 cups crisp basil leaves, washed and tapped dry

½ cup extra-virgin olive oil

3–4 cloves of garlic

1/3 cup pine nuts

¼ teaspoon salt

¼ teaspoon pepper (discretionary)

Procedure all fixings in a nourishment processor until smooth.

Serves 4

Preparation

Pesto shouldn't be made with basil; you can utilize cilantro, spinach, or on the other hand parsley. You could even do a blend of two unique herbs for assortment. For instance, utilize 2 cups basil with 2 cups spinach. You could likewise take a stab at utilizing various nuts, for example, pecans or walnuts.

Cashew Cabbage

The cashews make the flavor very appealing.

Ingredients

1 small head of cabbage, chopped

2 stalks of celery

½ medium onion, chopped

Sea salt to taste

Pepper to taste

½ cup rice milk or soy milk (more or less, as needed)

1 cup ground cashews

Preparation

Preheat oven to 350₃ F. Mix together cabbage, celery, onion, and seasonings, and place in a baking dish. Add rice milk or soy milk to cover; don't add too much. Bake until softened, about 50 minutes.

Top with ground cashews.

Delicious Green Beans with Garlic

Ingredients

I set up this dish frequently. It is simple, fast, and constantly a group pleaser.

3 garlic cloves, minced or squeezed

1 tablespoon in addition to 1 teaspoon olive oil

1 pound green beans, washed and cut

¼ cup sifted water

1 tablespoon in addition to 1 teaspoon tamari

2 teaspoons crude nectar

Preparation

In an enormous skillet, sauté the garlic in olive oil over medium warmth for about 3 minutes.

Include the green beans, water, tamari, and nectar, and cook over medium-low warmth until beans are delicate yet at the same time marginally firm. On the off chance that the water vanishes too rapidly, continue including water by the tablespoon—just enough to keep the beans steaming.

Serves 4

French Fries

Ingredients

1 pound yucca root

Sea salt to taste

Pepper to taste

Preparation

Steam or bake yucca roots until tender, about 40 minutes. When the yucca roots are nearly finished steaming, heat the oven to 375F. Allow yucca roots to cool enough so you can handle them. Cut off the outer waxy portion, and cut them into short sticks about inch thick.

Place on a baking pan, add salt and pepper (and other seasonings, as desired), and bake until they reach the desired crispiness.

Guacamole

Ingredients

It tastes so great with practically any dish. My preferred backups are rice saltines, plates of mixed greens, rice and beans, poached natural eggs, or sans wheat, sans corn burrito wraps.

3 ready avocados

2 garlic cloves, minced

2 tablespoons lemon juice

Ocean salt to taste

Pepper to taste

2–3 tablespoons new cilantro, minced (discretionary)

1 teaspoon without wheat tamari (discretionary; this will include salt, accordingly decrease or prohibit ocean salt)

½–1 little onion, minced (discretionary)

Preparation

Crush avocados with lemon juice. Include remaining fixings and blend well. In the event that you enable it to sit for ẁ hour, the preferences truly meet up.

Serves 6

Nut 'n' Curry Hummus

Ingredients

This is another dipping sauce; it is the best-tasting hummus. Using almond butter instead of peanut butter leaves nothing to be desired.

3 cups cooked garbanzo beans (2 cans)

¼ cup liquid from garbanzo beans

1/3 cup tahini (a sesame seed paste that can be purchased at most

Health-food stores)

3 garlic cloves, minced or pressed

¼ cup plus 1 tablespoon fresh lemon juice

3 tablespoons filtered water

½–1 teaspoon sea salt, or to taste

½ cup almond butter

2 teaspoons curry powder

Paprika for garnish

Parsley for garnish

Preparation

Blend all ingredients in blender until smooth.

Garnish with parsley and paprika, and serve with rice crackers, non-wheat bread, or fresh dipping vegetables such as carrots and celery. Depending on the moisture it tastes so great with practically any dish. My preferred backups are rice wafers, plates of mixed greens, rice and beans, poached natural eggs, or sans wheat, without corn burrito wraps.

3 ready avocados

2 garlic cloves, minced content of your almond spread and tahini, you may need to include some additional water or lemon juice for mixing.

Serves 6–8

Chikwizz

Ingredients

2 tablespoons lemon juice

Ocean salt to taste

Pepper to taste

2–3 tablespoons crisp cilantro, minced (discretionary)

1 teaspoon sans wheat tamari (discretionary; this will include salt, consequently lessen or prohibit ocean salt)

½–1 little onion, minced (discretionary)

Preparation

Include remaining fixings and blend well. On the off chance that you enable it to sit for hour, the preferences truly meet up.

Serves 6

Lemon Vegetable Rice

Ingredients

Light side dish that goes well with any dinner.

Juice of 2 medium lemons

2 tablespoons maple syrup

2½ cups of organic chicken broth

1½ cups of short-grain brown rice

½ teaspoon sea salt

1 cinnamon stick

5 whole cloves

2 tablespoons olive oil

1 teaspoon cumin seeds

1 small onion, thinly sliced

2 small zucchinis, sliced

1/3 cup roasted cashews, whole

2 tablespoons fresh sweet basil, chopped

Lemon wedges for garnish

Preparation

Pour lemon juice, maple syrup, and chicken broth into a saucepan; add rice, sea salt, cinnamon stick, and cloves.

Cover, bring to a boil, and boil for 2 minutes. Reduce heat and simmer for 25–30 minutes or until all liquid has been absorbed.

In a large skillet, saute cumin seeds in olive oil until they begin to pop. Add onion and cook for another 5 minutes over medium heat.

Add zucchini and cashews, and saute until zucchini is tender.

Stir in the basil and the rice, heat for another minute or two, and serve garnished with lemon wedges.

Serves 6–8

Mango Salsa

Of all the tomato dishes, salsa proved the hardest one for me to give up; therefore I had to come up with an alternative. You can use this version to replace salsa in any dish and to add a whole new dimension of flavor.

It's perfect over a mildly seasoned white fish such as halibut. It also can complement guacamole or any Mexican dish.

Ingredients

3 ripe mangos, peeled and diced

1 red onion, minced

4 tablespoons finely chopped cilantro

Juice of ½ lemons

1–2 medium-spice peppers, such an Anaheim peppers (depending on your tolerance for spice)

Sea salt to taste

1 medium red bell pepper, minced (optional)

Preparation

Combine all ingredients in a large bowl. Serve immediately with rice crackers, or store in the refrigerator. After it sits in the refrigerator for a little while, it tastes even better.

Serves 6–8

Alternatives

You can experiment with adding anything you want, e.g., black beans, green bell peppers, avocado. You can even try adding other fruit such as kiwis or nectarines. If you cannot tolerate spice, leave out the hot peppers; it still tastes great.

Mashed "Potatoes" (Mashed Artichokes)

If you desire mashed potatoes at your Thanksgiving dinner, this is a great alternative.

Ingredients

1 pound Jerusalem artichokes, scrubbed

1 tablespoon olive oil

1 tablespoon fresh tarragon, chopped

2 tablespoons soy milk

Sea salt and pepper to taste

Preparation

Preheat oven to 400 F.

Cut artichokes into wedges, hurl with olive oil, and spot in a preparing container. Prepare for 35–40 minutes or until delicate.

Expel from stove, crush well or go through a nourishment processor, furthermore, include remaining fixings. Mix again and serve warm.

Serves 6

Milk Thistle Seasoning Salt

This mix is a delicious—and more advantageous—choice to plain salt.

Ingredients

3 tablespoons milk thorn seeds (you can discover these at a wellbeing nourishment store)

3 tablespoons ocean salt

Crush the milk thorn seeds in an espresso processor until you have a fine powder.

Blend with ocean salt. Use as a trade for normal salt.

Preparation

Including dried kelp will manage the cost of much more supplements. Simply pound the kelp in the espresso processor and add the powder to the above blend.

Milk thorn is explicit in treating the liver, spleen, and kidneys. It is a powerful protectant of the liver and is shown for frail veins, blood balance, and liver ailments. The liver is a significant organ of detoxification.

Olive Oil–Butter Spread

Use it as a spread rather than plain natural margarine or on the other hand in cooking instead of plain natural olive oil.

Ingredients

1 pound natural spread, relaxed

1 cup extra-virgin olive oil

Preparation

In the event that important, heat the spread a tad to facilitiate the mixing of the fixings. Blend well.

Store in ice, and use sparingly as a spread.

Substitutions

Rather than olive oil you can utilize flaxseed oil or high-omega-3 oil, be that as it may, in the event that you do, abstain from warming it to high warmth, for example, for sautéing vegetables.

For sautéing, simply utilize olive oil or coconut oil.

"Peanut" Sauce

Peanut sauce is a favorite accompaniment with Thai dishes such as salad rolls and sate skewers. Using almonds instead of peanuts loses none of the savory goodness. Red curry paste and fish sauce are available in

Ingredients

5 ounces roasted, unsalted almonds

4 cups unsweetened coconut milk

2 tablespoons red curry paste

1 tablespoon honey

3 tablespoons lemon juice

3 teaspoons fish sauce

Preparation

Blend the nuts in a coffee grinder, in small batches, until they are the consistency of fine meal.

In a large skillet, combine ⅓ of the coconut milk with the curry paste; cook over high heat until the mixture separates.

Then reduce heat, add the remaining ingredients plus the rest of the coconut milk, and heat over medium heat for 15–20 minutes, stirring occasionally.

Remove from heat and allow sitting for 20 minutes before serving.

Serves 20

Substitutions

You could try other roasted nuts instead of almonds. This recipe is easily cut in half to make a smaller amount of sauce. If this version is too spicy, reduce the amount of red curry paste.

Salad Rolls

Ingredients

A favorite at Southeast Asian restaurants, such as those serving Thai or Vietnamese cuisine, salad rolls are deceptively simple to make.

10 sheets of round rice paper (found in Asian section of the grocery store)

Small package of rice noodles, cooked and rinsed

1 bunch of cilantro, minced or whole, with stems removed

½ pound of raw firm tofu, cut into long, thin strips

2 medium carrots, cut into long, thin strips

½ cucumber (cut lengthwise), cut into long, thin strips

Small amount of green leaf lettuce, shredded

Preparation

Cut cilantro, tofu, carrots, cucumber, and lettuce as directed, and make a pile of each for assembly.

Cook rice noodles according to package; rinse well with cold water also, put in a safe spot.

Fill a huge pot 1/2 inch to 1 inch deep with separated water and warmth over medium warmth. Plunge one sheet of rice paper into the water until it relaxes (around 15–20 seconds). Expel from water, enable overabundance water to deplete off, and move to a cutting board.

Each fixing in turn, orchestrate a modest quantity of rice noodles, cilantro, tofu, carrots, cucumbers, and lettuce on the base portion of the sheet of rice paper. Crease in the sides of the rice paper, and after that fold firmly into an enormous roll and put in a safe spot. Rehash with every one of the ten sheets of rice paper. You will figure out the amount of every fixing fits into each move by testing. Cut each move down the middle to uncover within.

Serve promptly with sans wheat tamari or "Nut" Sauce.

Serves 10

Alternatives

You can make these as basic or unpredictable as you want. Test with various vegetables, or even include extra fish. Including new mint rather than cilantro additionally gives a fresh, reviving taste.

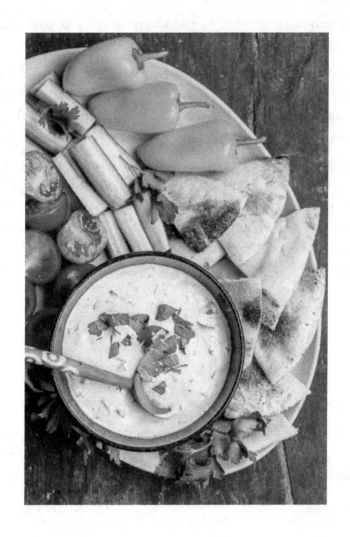

Scrumptious Green Beans

Straightforward green beans never tasted so great. This dish offers an extraordinary method to get some green vegetables into your relatives' diets.

Ingredients

2 tablespoons olive oil

½ teaspoon dark or yellow mustard seeds, accessible in the mass herb area of most wellbeing nourishment stores

½-inch 3D square of stripped ginger, cut julienne slim

¼ cup water

1 pound green beans, washed and cut

½ teaspoon ground cumin

¼ teaspoon turmeric

1 teaspoon ocean salt

2 tablespoons minced new cilantro

Juice of 1 lemon

Preparation

Saute mustard seeds and ginger in olive oil over moderate warmth until mustard seeds start to pop.

Include the beans and pan fried food over medium warmth for around 5 minutes.

Include the water, spread firmly, and stew for 5 minutes.

Expel the cover when the vast majority of the water has vanished. Include all remaining fixings aside from lemon squeeze, and keep cooking until the beans are warm yet at the same time marginally firm.

Include the lemon squeeze just before serving. Serve warm.

Serves 6

Substitutions

If you have parsley on hand, try that instead. Use this recipe with many different vegetables, for example asparagus, sliced carrots, or root vegetables cut into long, thin strips. Remember, green beans also taste great steamed, without any seasonings. Try them prepared that way if you haven't already.

Simple and Delectable Beets

Beets are so sweet that they really need no seasonings. But if you want to experiment with some new flavors, try this recipe.

Ingredients

3 beets, peeled and steamed until tender, but still slightly crunchy

1 teaspoon lemon juice

1 teaspoon honey (optional)

Sea salt and pepper to taste

Preparation

Steam beets and set aside to cool slightly.

Mix lemon juice and honey together over low heat in a 2-quart saucepan until well blended.

Turn off heat, slice beets, and add them to the pan. Mix gently.

Add sea salt and pepper to taste, and serve immediately.

If you are omitting the honey, just slice the cooked beets, sprinkle with lemon juice, sea salt, and pepper, and serve.

Serves 4

Substitutions

Use a dash of nutmeg or a bit of ginger instead of the honey to add flavor but no sugar.

Steamed Vegetables

Steamed vegetables are the ideal accompaniment to many dinners. The combination of brown rice and steamed vegetables has become a popular Japanese-style quick food, called *bento*. Find a favorite anti-inflammatory sauce and serve it with brown rice and steamed vegetables. Here are some guidelines for steaming:

45 Minutes

Beets, carrots, turnips, winter squash, artichokes

25 Minutes

Sweet potatoes, broccoli stalks, peas, parsnips, celery

15 Minutes

Garlic, cabbage, sweet peppers, cauliflower, onions, green beans, asparagus

7 Minutes

Mushrooms, broccoli tips, zucchini, summer squash

Preparation

Cut vegetables and place in steamer; cook for suggested length of time.

Remove from heat, season, and serve warm.

Note: Using an electric steamer with a timer is best, because you can pay attention to your other cooking duties as your vegetables are steaming. If you do not have an electric steamer, use a metal steamer basket that fits into a saucepan or large pot; add an inch or so of water beneath it. This allows the vegetables to remain out of the water while cooking. If you do not have anything in which to steam vegetables, add a small amount of water to a saucepan or soup pot (enough water to cover the bottom), add the vegetables, and steam them over medium heat. You may have to add water as it evaporates, so be sure to watch closely to keep the vegetables from burning.

Sweet Potato "Fries"

Ingredients

3 unpeeled sweet potatoes or yams, sliced into strips

1 teaspoon olive oil

Sea salt and pepper to taste

Dash of thyme

Dash of nutmeg

Preparation

Preheat oven to 400 degrees F. Toss olive oil, sweet potatoes, sea salt, and pepper in a large bowl.

Transfer to a baking pan, sprinkle with nutmeg and thyme, and bake for 30–35 minutes or until tender.

Serves 4

Substitutions

Many different seasonings will work with sweet potatoes. Experiment with allspice, rosemary, or grated orange zest.

Breads, Muffins, and Tortillas

Hannah's Rice-Flour Bread

Honey Millet Muffins

Spelt Bread

Spelt Tortillas

The All-Forgiving Banana Bread

Zucchini Bread

Hannah's Rice-Flour Bread

Gluten-free bread has never tasted so good. Try this one; you won't be disappointed.

Ingredients

½ cup warm water

2 teaspoons plus ¼ cup honey

4 teaspoons dry yeast granules

2 cups rice flour

2 cups tapioca flour

4 teaspoons xanthan gum, available in health-food stores

1½ teaspoons sea salt

1¼ cups soy milk

4 tablespoons melted organic butter

1 teaspoon vinegar

3 organic eggs, gently beaten

Preparation

In a small bowl, mix together water, 2 teaspoons honey, and yeast; set aside for 15 minutes.

In a large mixing bowl, combine dry ingredients.

Add wet ingredients to dry ingredients, and stir 20 times.

Add yeast mixture, and mix all with a mixer/beater. Note: Finished batter looks more like a thick cake batter than bread dough.

Divide batter into 2 equal amounts. Place in two 8 x 4 x 2⅝-inch, parchment paper–lined loaf pans. Smooth tops with a wet rubber spatula, and let rise in a warm place for approximately 1 hour.

Once dough has risen, preheat oven to 350₅ F. Bake loaves for 20–25 minutes.

Serves 6

Substitutions

You can experiment with different flours for this bread. You can also use any alternative milk in place of the soy milk. Coconut oil will easily replace the butter for those who can't tolerate any dairy.

Honey Millet Muffins

These little muffins can be served as a dessert because they taste so sweet.

Ingredients

1 organic egg

3 tablespoons organic butter, melted

½ cup milk substitute (e.g., soy milk) or water

½ cup honey

2 cups oat flour

1 teaspoon baking powder

½ teaspoon soda

½ teaspoon sea salt

1 cup millet, uncooked

½ teaspoon guar gum

Preparation

Preheat oven to 375 F. Mix all wet ingredients together in a large bowl.

Still mixing, add the dry ingredients slowly. Add millet last, and stir through the mixture.

Spoon mixture into muffin tin (greased if you are not using paper liners), and bake for 17–20 minutes.

Substitutions

This recipe contains enough guar gum to substitute for the gluten in wheat flour, so experiment with substituting different gluten-free flours. Oat happens to be my favorite because it tastes similar to whole wheat.

Spelt Bread

Because spelt has gluten in it, this bread has no problem binding together without an additional binder. Use this as a substitute for wheat bread, but avoid eating it every day because of its gluten content and its allergic potential.

Ingredients

1 tablespoon active dry yeast

1¼ cups warm filtered water

2 tablespoons organic coconut oil, warmed to a liquid consistency

3 tablespoons raw honey or brown rice syrup

1½ teaspoon sea salt

3½–4½ cups spelt flour (final amount used will depend on humidity)

Preparation

Mix in cup of warm water with yeast and let sit while preparing other ingredients.

In a large mixing bowl, mix 1 cup warm water, liquefied coconut oil, honey, salt, and 1½ cups of flour. When the yeast is bubbly, add it to the mixing bowl. Beat generously for at least 60 seconds to develop the gluten. Add another cup of flour gradually while stirring the mixture to make soft dough.

On a floured cutting board, knead the dough for 10 minutes while gradually adding more flour to form the dough into a round loaf. Add enough flour to keep the dough from sticking to the board but not so much that it falls apart. Avoid overworking the dough, which can lead to toughness.

When the loaf is finished, form it into a rectangle, place it in a greased bread pan, and set it in a warm place (85° F) to rise for 1 hour.

When the dough has risen slightly, bake at 350° F for 30 minutes.

Remember, the spelt flour will cause the bread to rise less than it would with wheat flour; thus the loaf will be more dense than you are used to.

Makes one small loaf

Substitutions

You can add some baking powder to this recipe to help the bread rise a little more, but don't overdo it: ¼ to 1/2 teaspoon is plenty. If you want to shape the dough into buns, divide the loaf into 10 parts and shape them any way you desire before allowing them to rise. You can try different combinations of flours, but remember, if the flour does not contain gluten, you also need to add a binder.

Spelt Tortillas

Tortillas can be served with many meals in place of bread or crackers. This wheat-free, corn-free version is fun to make and tastes great.

Ingredients

2 cups spelt flour (option: 1 cup white spelt flour, 1 cup whole-grain spelt flour)

1 cup warm filtered water (slightly more or less depending on humidity level)

2 tablespoons olive oil

¼ cup spelt flour (for rolling out the dough)

Preparation

Add water to spelt flour; knead the dough into a uniform mixture with your hands. Form the mixture into 8 egg-sized balls; set aside for about 20 minutes.

On a generously floured surface, use a rolling pin to roll out 1 ball into a circle. If the dough sticks to the rolling pin or the surface, add a little more flour. If it falls apart, add a few drops of water. Keep rolling the dough until you make a round, very thin tortilla. (As you become more practiced, you will find it easier to make a round shape; it is okay if your tortillas are not perfect the first time around.) Heat a skillet over medium-high heat, and add ¼ teaspoon olive oil. Place the tortilla in the skillet, and heat it just enough to lightly brown the bottom (about 60 seconds). When the tortilla is done on one side, it will begin to puff up. Flip the tortilla and heat briefly on the other side until lightly browned (about 60 more seconds). Place directly into a napkin and fold the napkin over it to keep it warm. Repeat with each dough ball. Serve immediately.

The All-Forgiving Banana Bread

You could do a lot to this recipe and still have it turn out great. Most people have no idea that it doesn't contain wheat. Compared to a regular banana bread recipe, it calls for only half the amount of butter/oil because it uses honey instead of sugar. It also contains half the amount of "sugar" of a regular banana bread.

Ingredients

¼ cup organic butter or vegan margarine (without hydrogenated oils), softened

1/8 cup organic coconut oil, warmed to a liquid consistency

½ cup honey

4 medium ripe bananas, puréed or thoroughly mashed with a fork

2 organic eggs

1 teaspoon baking soda

¼ teaspoon sea salt

1½ cup chopped walnuts

2 cups spelt flour

Preparation

Preheat oven to 375F.

Mix all wet ingredients together. You can use a blender to pure the bananas with the other wet ingredients. Gradually add the dry ingredients to the blender, and mix until smooth.

Pour into a 9 x 4 x 3-inch greased loaf pan or two small loaf pans.

Bake for 15 minutes; reduce oven to 350 F and bake for another 40–45 minutes.

Substitutions

As always, brown rice syrup is an acceptable substitute for honey. Plus, you can use pretty much any flour, or a combination of flours, and this recipe will turn out. Bananas add so much binder that they eliminate the need for the extra binder often called for when using non-wheat flour. The best option is to use a combination of rice flour, garbanzo flour, and oat flour. Other options include rye flour and tapioca flour. As for the nuts, you can also experiment with pecans, cashews, pumpkin seeds, sunflower seeds, flaxseeds, coconut, or just about anything else you have in the cupboard. A small amount of raisins will add extra sweetness.

The best variation is to use 1 cup of coconut and 1 cup millet in place of the nuts; then pour the batter into muffin pans. Follow the baking directions in the recipe for honey millet muffins.

Zucchini Bread

You really can't taste the difference between the old version and the healthy version of Zucchini bread.

Ingredients

¾ cup organic coconut oil, warmed to liquid consistency

3 organic eggs, beaten

2 cups grated zucchini

1 cup raw honey

1 teaspoon vanilla extract

3 cups oat flour

1 teaspoon baking soda

½ teaspoon sea salt

Preparation

Preheat oven to 350° F.

Mix together all wet ingredients, including zucchini. Gradually add dry ingredients, mixing thoroughly. Pour batter into a greased 9 x 4 x 3- inch loaf pan.

Bake for 1 hour or until a knife inserted in the center comes out clean.

Substitutions

You can try different combinations of flours with this recipe, but remember, if the flour does not contain gluten, you also need to add a binder.

Also experiment with adding seeds, chopped nuts, raisins, etc., for more texture and varied flavor.

Ircey Rice

If you have leftover, cooked brown rice in your refrigerator, this is an easy meal, especially on those mornings when you think there's nothing in your kitchen for breakfast. Always make sure to have nuts, seeds, and raisins on hand for baked goods; therefore, always have the ingredients to make this simple breakfast.

Ingredients

1 cup leftover cooked brown rice

¼ teaspoon cinnamon powder

1/8 cup raisins

½ teaspoon maple syrup (optional)

¼ cup chopped walnuts

¼ cup sunflower seeds

½ cup rice milk or other alternative milk

¼ teaspoon carob powder (optional)

Preparation

Combine all ingredients in a saucepan on the stove. Add milk to cover the rice for a cereal consistency. Warm over moderate heat to desired temperature and serve.

Serves 2

Substitutions

Any seeds and nuts will do. Experiment with whatever is in your cabinet.

Pumpkin spice or nutmeg would also be tasty. Or add fresh, cut fruit. You can always cook your rice fresh instead of using leftover rice, but the preparation time becomes longer than 5 minutes. Adding coconut milk instead of rice milk is a good way to add more fat to the diet and adds richer flavor.

Granulara

This simple-to-make version of an old favorite allows you to avoid the additives and hydrogenated oils that are found in most commercially processed granola.

Ingredients

6 cups rolled oats

1¼ cups unsweetened coconut

1 cup chopped almonds

1 cup raw, shelled sunflower seeds

½ cup sesame seeds

½ cup honey

½ cup organic coconut oil

Preparation

Preheat oven to 325° F.

Mix dry ingredients together in a large bowl.

Combine honey and oil in a saucepan and heat to a liquid consistency.

Pour over dry ingredients. Mix well. Flatten into a baking pan.

Bake for 15–20 minutes. Cool and store in an airtight container.

Serve with milk substitute and/or fresh fruit.

Serves 14

Substitutions

You can prepare this recipe with many different nuts and seeds and even dried fruit if you are not diabetic. For a change I sometimes add ¼ cup of almond butter or tahini. You can also try brown rice syrup instead of honey.

Protein Power Breakfast

This quick and easy breakfast is filled with many nutrients, including essential fatty acids and protein.

Ingredients

1 tablespoon flaxseeds

2 tablespoons sesame seeds

2 tablespoons sunflower seeds

1 teaspoon honey

½ medium banana, sliced

Preparation

Grind all seeds together in your coffee grinder (which by now must be going through an identity crisis). Place seeds in a cereal bowl. Add honey and a small amount of hot water or hot milk substitute. Mix together and top with sliced bananas. Sprinkle a little more honey or maple syrup on top and enjoy.

Serves 1

Substitutions

According to taste, you can use different combinations of seeds. I also like to add ground coconut. For a cold version of the breakfast, substitute cold milk in place of the hot water.

Oats

This morning meal takes less than three minutes to get ready. For an in a hurry rendition, utilize a glass bowl with a firmly fixed top, place every one of the fixings in it, and add it to the substance of your attaché or rucksack. In the event that you've utilized bubbling water, when you get the opportunity to work or school, your oat will be cool enough to eat.

Ingredients

1 cup nut-and-organic product muesli (characteristic without any added substances)

½–1 cup hot or bubbling water

½ teaspoon maple syrup (discretionary; the organic product in the oat includes sweetness)

Preparation

Mix all fixings together in an oat bowl.

Serves 1

Substitutions

Another brisk thought for hot oat is in any case 1 cup plain cereal, include a couple of solidified berries and somewhat nectar, and pour bubbling water over the blend. The water will liquefy the berries, preparing the cereal to eat in around 60 seconds. Adding ground flaxseeds to your cereal increments the fiber, protein, and basic fatty acids.

Wheat-Free Pancakes

This formula originates from an associate who has remarkable ability in the cooking expressions.

Ingredients

½ cup pecans, ground in nourishment processor to a fine powder

¾ cup spelt flour

¾ cup rice flour

1 teaspoon cream of tartar

1 teaspoon heating pop

¾ teaspoon ocean salt

11/3 cup water

1 tablespoon olive oil

Preparation

Discretionary—sprinkle crisp berries, slashed apple, or cleaved nuts into player.

Join ground pecans, flours, salt, cream of tartar, heating pop, and salt in a medium-sized blending bowl, mixing great.

Whisk 1 cup of water into dry fixings, at that point bit by bit include the rest of the water to arrive at wanted consistency. Include more water if the player is still excessively thick. Mix in any discretionary fixings until simply consolidated.

Brush or shower an enormous skillet or iron with modest quantity of oil.

Warmth skillet or iron over medium warmth. Drop player onto hot cooking surface utilizing a huge spoon. Cook the hotcake until air pockets structure on top; flip. Cook on the second side until gently seared.

Serves 6.

Substitutions

You can attempt different nuts (e.g., walnuts) and different kinds of flour. In the event that you supplant the spelt flour with non-gluten flour, you may need to include ⅛–¼ teaspoon guar gum or a mixed banana.

Simple Pancakes

These hotcakes, which have a delectable nutty flavor, offer a high measure of fiber and can be made with for all intents and purposes no flour.

Ingredients

3 tablespoons crude sunflower seeds, ground fine

3 tablespoons crude pumpkin seeds, ground fine

3 natural eggs

¼ cup non-gluten oat flour (any non-wheat or non-gluten flour will do)

¼ cup rice milk

¼ cup blueberries (discretionary)

Preparation

Consolidate all fixings in a medium-sized bowl and blend well until clusters have broken down.

Empty hitter into 3-inch distance across hovers in the container. At the point when hotcakes start to air pocket, flip and cook on the opposite side for a short measure of time until gently sautéed on the two sides.

Serves 2

Substitutions

You may add berries or other organic product to this formula. In the event that the natural product is solidified, the hitter tends to bunch around it; the hotcakes still end up great. Ben Unterserher, a back rub specialist in McMinnville, Oregon, changed over this formula into astonishing level bread that is like pita bread. He included

Eggnog

This is a simple breakfast to whip together for yourself or your kids and offers a decent wellspring of complete protein in the first part of the day.

Ingredients

2 natural eggs

1 cup rice milk, chilled

1 tablespoon vanilla concentrate

Run cinnamon

Run nutmeg

Preparation

Consolidate all fixings in an enormous cup or bowl, and blend well until blend looks uniform.

Strain blend through little strainer into a serving glass and serve.

Serves 1

Substitutions

Soy milk or substitute milk can be utilized instead of rice milk.

Smoothie

This quick, basic breakfast can support your glucose until midmorning or lunch.

Ingredients

2 tablespoons soy protein powder

1 cup natural solidified berries (blueberries, strawberries, raspberries, blackberries, fruits)

2 cups soy milk (use water in the event that you like, or half water and half milk)

Spot all fixings in blender and mix to wanted thickness and consistency.

Serves 1–2

Preparation

When you get its hang, you can make a smoothie in less than five minutes, move it to a container or mug, and be out the entryway, nearly as fast as though you'd skipped breakfast. Set aside a few minutes; it is justified, despite all the trouble.

Substitutions

You can utilize a rice-based protein powder, or, rather than protein powder, you can utilize 1/2 square or a greater amount of smooth tofu. Additionally, you can utilize any milk substitute (e.g., rice milk, almond milk).

You may include the accompanying fixings based your taste buds and your dietary needs.

Home grown "Juice"

This tea is an amazing substitution for natural product juice. Each youngster adores juice; what's more, here is a substitute without all the additional sugars. Furthermore, the hibiscus makes it a quite red. Regardless of whether you improve the tea a smidgen, it will still be more beneficial than locally acquired juice. Your children won't know the distinction!

All fixings ought to be accessible in the mass area of a well-supplied characteristic nourishments store.

Ingredients

½ cup dried crataegus (hawthorn) leaves

½ cup dried crataegus (hawthorn) berries

½ cup rose hips

¼ cup dried hibiscus blossoms

½ cup dried peppermint leaves

Get-up-and-go of 1 medium lemon

Nectar to taste (discretionary)

Preparation

Combine all fixings and store in a sealed shut holder for use as required. For each serving, utilize 1 tablespoon of tea blend and 10 liquid ounces (11/2 cup) of sifted water. For a gallon of tea (roughly 12 servings), utilize a gallon of separated water and 12 tablespoons (3/4 cup) of tea blend.

In a tea pot (for little quantities) or a huge pot, carry water to a bubble. Expel from heat, include dried herbs and lemon pizzazz, and permit to soak for 10–15 minutes.

Channel into a huge compartment through an exceptionally fine strainer or 2–3 thicknesses of cheesecloth. At the point when tea is still warm, add nectar to taste what's more, store in icebox. Serve chilled (or, on the off chance that you want, warm).

Yield: 21/2 cup dried tea blend, or roughly 36 servings.

Chai

Ingredients

3 cups rice milk

3 cups water

1 cinnamon sticks, 2 inches long

8 whole black peppercorns

2 whole cloves

4 cardamom seeds

½ teaspoon whole cumin seeds

¼ teaspoon ground allspice

1/8 teaspoon ground nutmeg

Serves 6

Preparation

Combine all fixings and store in a sealed shut holder for use as required. For each serving, utilize 1 tablespoon of tea blend and 10 liquid ounces (11/2 cup) of sifted water. For a gallon of tea (roughly 12 servings), utilize a gallon of separated water and 12 tablespoons (3/4 cup) of tea blend.

In a tea pot (for little quantities) or a huge pot, carry water to a bubble. Expel from heat, include dried herbs and lemon pizzazz, and permit to soak for 10–15 minutes.

Channel into a huge compartment through an exceptionally fine strainer or 2–3 thicknesses of cheesecloth. At the point when tea is still warm, add nectar to taste what's more, store in icebox. Serve chilled (or, on the off chance that you want, warm).

Yield: 21/2 cup dried tea blend, or roughly 36 servings.

Quieting Tea

Ingredients

2 sections chamomile blooms

1 section passionflower

1 section hypericum (St. John's wort)

1 section lavender blooms

Preparation

Combine all fixings and store in a sealed shut holder for use as required. For each serving, utilize 1 tablespoon of tea blend and 10 liquid ounces (11/2 cup) of sifted water. For a gallon of tea (roughly 12 servings), utilize a gallon of separated water and 12 tablespoons (3/4 cup) of tea blend.

In a tea pot (for little quantities) or a huge pot, carry water to a bubble. Expel from heat, include dried herbs and lemon pizzazz, and permit to soak for 10–15 minutes.

Channel into a huge compartment through an exceptionally fine strainer or 2–3 thicknesses of cheesecloth. At the point when tea is still warm, add nectar to taste what's more, store in icebox. Serve chilled (or, on the off chance that you want, warm).

Yield: 21/2 cup dried tea blend, or roughly 36 servings.

The Stress Reliever

Ingredients

2 sections oat straw

2 sections linden flower

1 section passionflower

1 section lemon demulcent

Preparation

Combine all fixings and store in a sealed shut holder for use as required. For each serving, utilize 1 tablespoon of tea blend and 10 liquid ounces (11/2 cup) of sifted water. For a gallon of tea (roughly 12 servings), utilize a gallon of separated water and 12 tablespoons (3/4 cup) of tea blend.

In a tea pot (for little quantities) or a huge pot, carry water to a bubble. Expel from heat, include dried herbs and lemon pizzazz, and permit to soak for 10–15 minutes.

Channel into a huge compartment through an exceptionally fine strainer or 2–3 thicknesses of cheesecloth. At the point when tea is still warm, add nectar to taste what's more, store in icebox. Serve chilled (or, on the off chance that you want, warm).

Yield: 21/2 cup dried tea blend, or roughly 36 servings.

Adrenal Support Tea

(For vitality)

1 section Siberian ginseng

1 section gout kola

1 section ginkgo biloba

1 section licorice

Preparation

Combine all fixings and store in a sealed shut holder for use as required. For each serving, utilize 1 tablespoon of tea blend and 10 liquid ounces (11/2 cup) of sifted water. For a gallon of tea (roughly 12 servings), utilize a gallon of separated water and 12 tablespoons (3/4 cup) of tea blend.

In a tea pot (for little quantities) or a huge pot, carry water to a bubble. Expel from heat, include dried herbs and lemon pizzazz, and permit to soak for 10–15 minutes.

Channel into a huge compartment through an exceptionally fine strainer or 2–3 thicknesses of cheesecloth. At the point when tea is still warm, add nectar to taste what's more, store in icebox. Serve chilled (or, on the off chance that you want, warm).

Yield: 21/2 cup dried tea blend, or roughly 36 servings.

Basic Mood Tea (to lift the spirits)

Ingredients

1 section passionflower

1 section lemon demulcent

1 section hypericum (St. John's wort)

Preparation

Combine all fixings and store in a sealed shut holder for use as required. For each serving, utilize 1 tablespoon of tea blend and 10 liquid ounces (11/2 cup) of sifted water. For a gallon of tea (roughly 12 servings), utilize a gallon of separated water and 12 tablespoons (3/4 cup) of tea blend.

In a tea pot (for little quantities) or a huge pot, carry water to a bubble. Expel from heat, include dried herbs and lemon pizzazz, and permit to soak for 10–15 minutes.

Channel into a huge compartment through an exceptionally fine strainer or 2–3 thicknesses of cheesecloth. At the point when tea is still warm, add nectar to taste what's more, store in icebox. Serve chilled (or, on the off chance that you want, warm).

Yield: 21/2 cup dried tea blend, or roughly 36 servings.

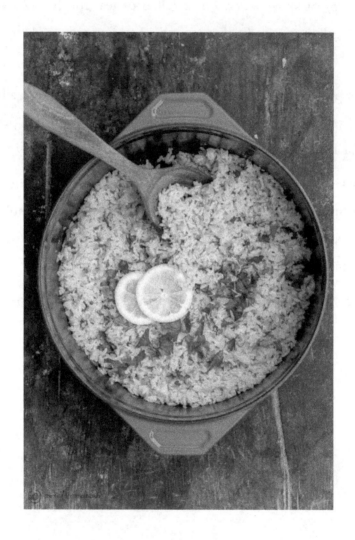

Purging Tea (No soaking vital)

Ingredients

Juice of ½ lemons

1 tablespoon unadulterated maple syrup

8–10 ounces sifted water, cold or hot

¼ teaspoon cayenne (decline on the off chance that you can't endure the zestiness)

Preparation

Combine all fixings and store in a sealed shut holder for use as required. For each serving, utilize 1 tablespoon of tea blend and 10 liquid ounces (11/2 cup) of sifted water. For a gallon of tea (roughly 12 servings), utilize a gallon of separated water and 12 tablespoons (3/4 cup) of tea blend.

In a tea pot (for little quantities) or a huge pot, carry water to a bubble. Expel from heat, include dried herbs and lemon pizzazz, and permit to soak for 10–15 minutes.

Channel into a huge compartment through an exceptionally fine strainer or 2–3 thicknesses of cheesecloth. At the point when tea is still warm, add nectar to taste what's more, store in icebox. Serve chilled (or, on the off chance that you want, warm).

Yield: 21/2 cup dried tea blend, or roughly 36 servings.

Detoxification Tea

Ingredients

1 section burdock root

1 section dandelion root

2 sections licorice root

Preparation

Combine all fixings and store in a sealed shut holder for use as required. For each serving, utilize 1 tablespoon of tea blend and 10 liquid ounces (11/2 cup) of sifted water. For a gallon of tea (roughly 12 servings), utilize a gallon of separated water and 12 tablespoons (3/4 cup) of tea blend.

In a tea pot (for little quantities) or a huge pot, carry water to a bubble. Expel from heat, include dried herbs and lemon pizzazz, and permit to soak for 10–15 minutes.

Channel into a huge compartment through an exceptionally fine strainer or 2–3 thicknesses of cheesecloth. At the point when tea is still warm, add nectar to taste what's more, store in icebox. Serve chilled (or, on the off chance that you want, warm).

Yield: 21/2 cup dried tea blend, or roughly 36 servings.

Tea to Relax the Nerves

Ingredients

1 section hibiscus blossoms

1 section basil

1 section catnip

1 section lemon ointment

2 sections peppermint

Preparation

Combine all fixings and store in a sealed shut holder for use as required. For each serving, utilize 1 tablespoon of tea blend and 10 liquid ounces (11/2 cup) of sifted water. For a gallon of tea (roughly 12 servings), utilize a gallon of separated water and 12 tablespoons (3/4 cup) of tea blend.

In a tea pot (for little quantities) or a huge pot, carry water to a bubble. Expel from heat, include dried herbs and lemon pizzazz, and permit to soak for 10–15 minutes.

Channel into a huge compartment through an exceptionally fine strainer or 2–3 thicknesses of cheesecloth. At the point when tea is still warm, add nectar to taste what's more, store in icebox. Serve chilled (or, on the off chance that you want, warm).

Yield: 21/2 cup dried tea blend, or roughly 36 servings.

Simple Digestion Tea

2 sections peppermint

1 section fennel

1 section anise seed

½ part gingerroot

Preparation

Combine all fixings and store in a sealed shut holder for use as required. For each serving, utilize 1 tablespoon of tea blend and 10 liquid ounces (11/2 cup) of sifted water. For a gallon of tea (roughly 12 servings), utilize a gallon of separated water and 12 tablespoons (3/4 cup) of tea blend.

In a tea pot (for little quantities) or a huge pot, carry water to a bubble. Expel from heat, include dried herbs and lemon pizzazz, and permit to soak for 10–15 minutes.

Channel into a huge compartment through an exceptionally fine strainer or 2–3 thicknesses of cheesecloth. At the point when tea is still warm, add nectar to taste what's more, store in icebox. Serve chilled (or, on the off chance that you want, warm).

Yield: 21/2 cup dried tea blend, or roughly 36 servings.

Resistant Booster Tea

2 sections elderberry

2 sections Echinacea

1 section licorice

1 section hyssop

1 section thyme

2 sections peppermint

Preparation

Combine all fixings and store in a sealed shut holder for use as required. For each serving, utilize 1 tablespoon of tea blend and 10 liquid ounces (11/2 cup) of sifted water. For a gallon of tea (roughly 12 servings), utilize a gallon of separated water and 12 tablespoons (3/4 cup) of tea blend.

In a tea pot (for little quantities) or a huge pot, carry water to a bubble. Expel from heat, include dried herbs and lemon pizzazz, and permit to soak for 10–15 minutes.

Channel into a huge compartment through an exceptionally fine strainer or 2–3 thicknesses of cheesecloth. At the point when tea is still warm, add nectar to taste what's more, store in icebox. Serve chilled (or, on the off chance that you want, warm).

Yield: 21/2 cup dried tea blend, or roughly 36 servings.

Drowsy Tea

2 sections chamomile

2 sections skullcap

1 section passion flower

1 section valerian (discretionary)

Directions

There are two distinct approaches to make teas: imbuement and decoction. Most teas are implantations, made when herbs are put in heated water and left to soak for around 15 minutes. A decoction is utilized when roots are included. For a decoction, the roots should be bubbled for a period previously soaking to draw out their restorative quality.

For a Decoction

Utilize 1 tablespoon tea mix for each 10 liquid ounces (1ʍ cup) of sifted water. In a pot or pot, place the root just (not different fixings) in water and heat to the point of boiling.

Spread, lessen warmth to medium, and enable the water to stew for 15–25 minutes.

Expel from the burner and enable the tea to soak an additional 10 minutes, secured. On the off chance that there are different herbs to mix with this tea, include them at this time.

Channel through a fine strainer or 2–3 thicknesses of cheesecloth.

Substitution Ideas

These tea mixes are not unchangeable; they're simply recommendations. I as a rule make teas dependent on what I have in my herb cabinet. In the event that I am absent a few fixings, I use others in their place. Keep in mind, you are the imaginative plan in your own kitchen. On the off chance that you need to include lemon pizzazz, hibiscus blooms, nectar, or different fixings to your teas to make them increasingly tasteful, feel free.

These teas are not restorative medicines and are not intended to replace therapeutic treatment.

Almond Milk

Almond milk, which is exceptionally easy to make, is better than bovine's milk in light of its diminished allergen potential and its noteworthy substance of plant-based basic fatty acids. At the point when you're lacking in time, you can purchase almond milk in the wellbeing nourishment segment of supermarkets or at any characteristic nourishments store.

Ingredients

1 cup crude, entire almonds

3 cups separated water (pretty much, contingent upon wanted taste and consistency)

Splash the almonds medium-term in a limited quantity of separated water.

Preparation

Channel off the water. Rub every almond between your fingers to evacuate the dark colored skin. Mix the cleaned almonds with a modest quantity of crisp separated water at a fast until they arrive at a smooth consistency.

Subsequent to mixing, add water to arrive at wanted taste and thickness. At that point, strain the milk through a fine strainer or two layers of cheesecloth. You may include sugar, yet it is generally not required on the off chance that you utilize crisp almonds.

Serves 4

Substitutions

In the event that you need to make the formula somewhat quicker and less difficult, use fragmented almonds, which don't have any strip to rub off in the wake of splashing.

You can make milk from various sorts of nuts. Not all nuts should be doused medium-term to evacuate the strip. Continuously start by mixing the nuts with a limited quantity of water, at that point adding more water to wanted taste and consistency.

Sesame Milk

This milk is jam-pressed with significant supplements and protein. It's an incredible method to get some sustenance into your kids. I like to blend a balance of sesame milk and rice milk for a heavenly drink on the stones.

Ingredients

1 cup sesame seeds

3½ cups sifted water

1 tablespoon nectar

2 teaspoons carob powder

Preparation

Pound the seeds in an espresso processor and join with residual fixings in an enormous compartment. Shake altogether, and let sit for 15 minutes. Shake again and strain through 2 thicknesses of cheesecloth or a fine strainer. Chill in the fridge or serve over ice. Keep refrigerated.

Serves 4

Chicken Curry Made Simple

It's ideal for those evenings when you would prefer not to spend a lot time in the kitchen. To make the activity considerably faster, hack the vegetables early. Serve over a most loved grain, for example, fragrant jasmine rice or on the other hand quinoa.

Ingredients

1 enormous onion, cleaved

3–4 cloves garlic, minced

1 tablespoon olive oil

5–6 carrots cut into sticks

1 14.5-ounce cans natural chicken stock

2–3 boneless, skinless natural chicken bosoms (about 1½ pounds meat), cubed

1 13.5-ounce would coconut be able to drain

Curry powder to taste

Ginger powder to taste

Preparation

In a huge pot, saute garlic and onions in half of the olive oil over medium warmth. Include carrots and keep sautéing. While carrots are cooking, in a different pan saute chicken in staying olive oil until done. To the pan with the vegetables, include chicken soup, coconut milk, and cooked chicken. Add curry powder and ginger to taste. (Utilize 2–4 teaspoons curry powder and 1–2 teaspoons ginger powder.) Continue to cook until flavors merge and sauce is warmed through, around 10 minutes.

Serves 5

Substitutions

You can add any vegetables you like to this flexible formula. Broccoli consistently makes a decent expansion to curries.

Extra Veggie Burgers

This is one of those plans that consistently come through after all other options have been exhausted. It turns out various unfailingly and changes your remains into something enjoyable to eat. Note: We did exclude nutritional data in light of the fact that the purpose of this formula is to try different things with whatever scraps you have close by.

Ingredients

1 cup extra cooked vegetables (pan-seared, steamed, and so forth.)

½ cup extra cooked darker rice, quinoa, and so forth., from earlier night

2 natural eggs, beaten

½ squashed banana (discretionary), as a coupling operator

Preparation

Preheat broiler to 375F.

Join all fixings in a blender; mix until the vegetables and grains are finely cleaved. Structure the blend into patties, and spot them on a lubed heating dish.

Another choice is to hack the extra veggies in a chopper or nourishment processor, and after that blend them with different fixings in a bowl, utilizing your hands. On the off chance that you don't have either a chopper or a blender, simply mince the vegetables by hand and blend them with the rest of the fixings.

You shouldn't have to season the burgers, in light of the fact that your supper from the night before will have just been prepared.

Serves 2

Substitutions

You can add such huge numbers of various things to these burgers. In the event that you can't endure eggs, use another cover from the substitutions table in the Appendix.

Turkey Meatloaf

This formula requires little planning time however needs an hour to heat. It is basic enough to get ready toward the beginning of the day and toss in the stove when you return home from work.

Ingredients

1 pound ground natural turkey

¼ cup milk substitute (or chicken or vegetable stock)

1 natural egg

½ cup finely cleaved onion

½ cup ground carrot

½ cup minced parsley or cilantro

¼ cup finely cleaved celery

½–1½ teaspoon onion powder

½–1½ teaspoon garlic powder

½–1½ teaspoon dried oregano

½–1½ teaspoon dried sage

½ teaspoon salt

¼–½ teaspoon pepper

Preparation

Preheat broiler to 350 F.

Blend all fixings in a bowl, making a point to mix well. (hand are the best method to get everything very much mixed, so make a plunge and have some good times.)

Put everything into a lubed 9 x 5-inch portion skillet.

Put on fire for 60 minutes. Channel squeezes and serve by the cut. Children will love it.

Serves 4

Substitutions

The quantities of flavors are given in ranges since certain individuals incline toward an increasingly delightful meatloaf; all things considered utilize the bigger quantity. On the off chance that you can't endure eggs, simply supplant the egg with 1/2 banana or other cover. Additionally include ground or entire flaxseeds, pumpkin seeds, or sunflower seeds.

Sodium Filled Grain

Grain has a great surface for soups and oat. Purchase non-pearled (unhulled) grain on the grounds that pearling evacuates in excess of 30 percent of the grain's sustenance.

Ingredients

1 cup grain

3 cups sifted water

Preparation

Spot water and grain in a 2-quart pan. Bring to bubble, decrease heat to low, spread, and stew for 1 hour and 15 minutes. On the other hand, place all fixings in a stewing pot and stew on high for around 3 hours. Yields 3 cups

Dark Colored Rice

One regularly utilize natural short-grain dark colored rice since it cooks quicker and I favor the surface. Dark colored rice is better than white rice from numerous points of view. It has 12 percent more protein, 33 percent more calcium, more B nutrients, furthermore, a greater amount of different supplements. I just utilize white rice for one dish: sushi. Dark colored rice can supplement most meals and it is useful for breakfast.

You can likewise add cooked dark colored rice to heated merchandise for additional surface, flavor, and dampness.

Ingredients

1 cup dark colored rice, short or long grain

2 cups separated water

Preparation

Spot water and rice in a 2- quart pot. Bring to bubble; quickly lessen warmth to low.

Serves 6

Millet Dish

Millet can be utilized instead of rice or quinoa. It adds a crunchy surface to servings of mixed greens and vegetable dishes.

Ingredients

1 cup millet

3 cups sifted water

Preparation

Spot water and millet in a2-quart pan. Bring to bubble, diminish warmth to low, spread, and stew for 35–40 minutes. Yields 31/2 cups

Serves 7

Local Oats

Oats are unfortunately underused. Don't simply consider them cereal. You can add them to soups and goulashes for some additional body, or to treats or other heated merchandise.

Ingredients

1 cup oats

2 cups sifted water

Preparation

Spot water and oats in a 2- quart pan. Cook over low warmth for 20–25 minutes.

Yields 13/4 cups

Serves 3

Quinoa

It is higher in protein than some other grain, and its protein is a complete protein, which means it contains the majority of the fundamental amino acids, a quality shared by not many plant-based nourishments.

Ingredients

1 cup quinoa

2 cups separated water

Preparation

Spot water and quinoa in a 2-quart pot. Bring to bubble and afterward right away diminish warmth to low.

Stew, secured, for 10–15 minutes or until all water has been assimilated.

Yields 21/2 cups

Serves 5

Curry Chicken Salad

Subsequent to appreciating a curry chicken plate of mixed greens sandwich in the shop of a health food store, I needed to think of a formula for it.

Ingredients

1¼ pounds natural chicken bosom, heated and cubed

½ cup natural mayonnaise (search for one with every single normal fixing)

½ cup diced celery

½ medium Fuji apple, diced

¼–½ cup raisins (preclude on the off chance that you are diabetic)

¼ cup diced onion (discretionary)

2½ teaspoons curry powder

½ teaspoon turmeric

½ teaspoon salt or to taste

Run of pepper

6 enormous lettuce leaves (for serving)

Preparation

Combine all fixings, and permit to sit in cooler for in any event

30 minutes. Serve on lettuce leaves.

Serves 4

Substitutions

For a veggie lover rendition, attempt 3D squares of firm prepared tofu rather than chicken.

Strawberry Spinach Salad

Ingredients

2 tablespoons sesame seeds

1 tablespoon poppy seeds

½ cup olive oil

¼ cup nectar

¼ cup red wine vinegar

¼ teaspoon paprika

¼ teaspoon mustard

1 tablespoon dried minced onion

¼ cup toasted, fragmented almonds

Preparation

In a huge bowl, join spinach, strawberries, and almonds.

Pour dressing over plate of mixed greens, hurl, and refrigerate 10–15 minutes prior serving.

Serves 4

Substitutions

Attempt this plate of mixed greens with avocados, different nuts (e.g., cashews, pecans, hazelnuts), what's more, organic products (e.g., blueberries, diced pear).

Delectable Lemon Vinaigrette Salad

Ingredient

¼ cup lemon juice

¼ cup olive oil or flaxseed oil

2 tablespoons balsamic vinegar

1 tablespoon unadulterated maple syrup

½ teaspoon red pepper drops

1 teaspoon dried basil

Preparation:

In a little skillet over medium warmth, toast pine nuts in a modest quantity of oil until brilliant dark colored. Hurl with lettuce leaves and olives.

In a different bowl, blend dressing. Pour over top of serving of mixed greens.

Serves 4.

Substitutions:

Flaxseed oil is constantly a solid substitute for olive oil in plates of mixed greens. Furthermore, other than exploring different avenues regarding various sorts of foods grown from the ground, you can attempt including ground crude carrots, radishes, or beets.

The Not-So-Greek Salad

Ingredients

½ cup cold-squeezed olive oil

½ cup crisp pressed lemon juice

4 cloves garlic, minced

1 teaspoon dried oregano

1 teaspoon dark pepper

1 teaspoon salt

Preparation

In a little skillet over medium warmth, toast pine nuts in a modest quantity of oil till brilliant dark colored.

Get ready serving of mixed greens by hurling greens with cucumbers, olives, and pine nuts. In a little bowl consolidate all dressing fixings and blend well. Pour over plate of mixed greens and serve right away.

Wipe Out-the-Refrigerator Soup

Ingredients

For the juices:

6 cups natural chicken stock

1 onion, minced

3 garlic cloves, minced or squeezed

2 tablespoons garlic bean sauce (from Asian area of grocery store)

2 tablespoons miso soup glue

Herbs, flavors, and ocean salt to taste

Preparation

The way in to a decent tasting soup is to get the juices directly before including vegetables or potentially meat. Prior to turning on the stove, taste the juices cold furthermore, alter the seasonings.

Start by joining chicken stock with onions and garlic in a soup pot.

Include herbs, flavors, garlic bean sauce, miso, or whatever else you want.

At the point when the taste meets your fulfillment, turn the burner to medium high, heat the soup to the point of boiling, at that point right away lessen warmth and stew for 15 minutes, secured. Continue tasting and including seasonings as wanted.

For a thicker stock, you can include ground oats as of now. Additionally include vegetables. Try not to utilize an excessive number of these fixings, since they are thick.

Include vegetables, and stew, secured, for an additional 15 minutes. Include extra meat and stew, secured, for another 15–30 minutes.

After the vegetables have cooked agreeable to you, turn off the heat and enable the soup to sit secured for in any event 15 minutes prior serving; this progression enables the flavors to blend. Serve plain or with rice wafers.

Serves 6

Substitutions

As referenced before, you can and should have a go at anything in this soup. Season the juices with tamari rather than or notwithstanding garlic bean sauce. Include a squeeze of dried herbs, for example, thyme, marjoram, or Herbs de Provence.

Use ground quinoa as a thickener rather than oats. Utilize split peas, grain, or then again naval force beans rather than lentils. Utilize remaining meat of any sort, including turkey or fish.

Minute Avocado Soup

This soup is anything but difficult to make, tastes extraordinary, and fills the stomach on a cool night.

Ingredients:

2 medium ready avocados

2 cups almond milk

½ teaspoon cumin

½ teaspoon ground ginger

½ teaspoon salt

1 clove garlic, minced

Preparation

Squash avocados in a container.

Include every single outstanding fixing. Mix well until blended completely. You may utilize an electric mixer or blender for this progression.

At the point when the soup is very much blended, heat only enough to serve.

Serves 4

Cream of Carrot and Ginger Soup

Ingredients

2 pounds natural carrots

6 garlic cloves

2 medium yellow onions

2 tablespoons olive oil

2 cups natural chicken juices

11/3 cups coconut milk

1/3 cup soy milk

2 teaspoons ground crisp ginger

½ teaspoon ocean salt

½ teaspoon pepper

2 tablespoons dried parsley (as topping)

Preparation

Steam the carrots until delicate.

While the carrots are steaming, sauté the garlic and onions in the olive oil until they are mollified and marginally dark colored in shading.

Consolidate steamed carrots, cooked garlic and onions, and all remaining fixings in a blender. Mix on the pure setting. (Alert: Don't heat the fluid fixings before mixing. Utilizing a blender to blend huge quantities of hot fluids can cause a fast development in the fluids, which can make a little blast! In the event that you need to mix hot fluids in a blender, do as such in a few little clusters.)

Warmth the mixed soup in a huge pan, and serve embellished with dried parsley.

Serves 6

Nutty Onion Soup

Ingredients:

1 quart of natural chicken soup

1½ cup separated water

2 cups cashews

2 little onions, hacked

3 tablespoons cold-squeezed, extra-virgin olive oil

2 teaspoons marjoram

2 teaspoons thyme

1 tablespoon chives, minced (for decorate)

Preparation

Pound the nuts in an espresso processor until fine.

Expel from warmth and permit to cool marginally.

Move the nuts and onions to a blender with outstanding fixings what's more, mix until smooth.

Move to a soup pot and stew on medium warmth for 20–30 minutes.

Serve warm, embellished with minced chives.

Serves 4

Coconut Vanilla "Dessert"

Ingredients

This formula requires a dessert creator.

1 13.5-ounce would coconut be able to drain

1¼ cup vanilla soy milk

¼ cup nectar

1 tablespoon vanilla concentrate

Preparation

Join all fixings in a medium-sized bowl; blend well until nectar is broken down.

Turn dessert producer on and pour blend in.

Give ice a chance to cream producer work for 30 minutes. Serve right away.

Serves 6

Solidified Bananas Food

These are the ideal summer treat. Make numerous on the double and keep them in the cooler for you or your youngsters at whatever point a sweet needing strikes.

On the off chance that you have something solid available, you are substantially less liable to gorge on nourishment that isn't beneficial for you.

Ingredients

1 ready banana, cut into thirds

1 tablespoon carob powder

¼ teaspoon water

½ teaspoon nectar

¼ cup unsweetened coconut, ground medium

Preparation

In a little pan over medium-low warmth, join carob powder and enough water to make glue. Include nectar and warmth to wanted consistency.

Ensure it isn't excessively runny.

Coat each bit of banana in carob blend and move in coconut.

Wrap exclusively and place in the cooler until totally solidified (at least 30 minutes).

Remove them from the cooler 20 minutes before serving.

Serves 1.

Ginger Snaps

Ginger snaps are an exceptionally pleasant mix of sound fixings with a palatable taste.

Ingredients

1½ cup custard flour

1 cup rye flour

½ teaspoon guar gum

1 teaspoon preparing powder

1 teaspoon preparing pop

½ teaspoon salt

¼ cup maple syrup

¼ cup darker rice syrup

½ cup coconut oil, warmed to a fluid consistency

5 tablespoons ground crisp ginger

Preparation

Preheat broiler to 350 F.

In an enormous bowl, mix together the flours, guar gum, heating powder, preparing pop, and salt. Include the maple syrup, darker rice syrup, oil, and ginger. Mix together delicately until simply blended. Scoop spoon-sized bits onto a delicately lubed treat sheet and heat for 12–15 minutes.

Generous Healthy Cookies

These treats were my first analysis with anti-inflammatory preparing. They have an extraordinary flavor and a great deal of fiber.

Ingredients:

1 natural egg, beaten

¼ cup rice milk

½ cup natural margarine (1 stick), relaxed

½ cup coconut oil, warmed to a fluid consistency

½ cup unadulterated nectar

1 teaspoon vanilla concentrate

1½ cups oat flour

1 teaspoon preparing pop

1 teaspoon cinnamon

1 teaspoon ocean salt

3 cups moved oats

½ cup pecan pieces

¼ cup sunflower seeds

½ cup minced, stripped apple

Preparation

Preheat broiler to 375F.

Combine wet fixings, including relaxed margarine, in an enormous bowl. In a different, littler bowl, combine flour, preparing pop, cinnamon, and ocean salt. Gradually add dry fixings to wet fixings, blending continually, until you have a smooth hitter. Include oats, nuts, seeds, and apple, blending tenderly until blend is uniform. Drop with a spoon onto a lubed treat sheet, and heat for 9–12 minutes.

Substitutions

In the event that you can't endure any dairy, coconut oil can be utilized rather than spread with no adjustment in enhance. Any nuts or seeds and numerous organic products can be utilized, so don't be hesitant to analyze. Add ground zucchini to soak and add flavor to these treats.

No-Bake Oatmeal Cookies

They are useful for exceptional events. It is smarter to eat these than to gorge on white flour, white sugar, or handled prepared products.

Ingredients

½ cup nectar

½ cup dark colored rice syrup

3 cups oats

3 teaspoons carob powder

2 teaspoons vanilla concentrate

¼ cup softened natural margarine (discretionary)

1 cup natural almond margarine

Preparation

Combine all fixings, structure into treat shapes, mastermind them on wax paper, and spot in fridge to cool. When treats have cooled, you can store them in a hermetically sealed holder in the cooler.

Substitutions

You can utilize 1 cup nectar or 1 cup dark colored rice syrup in the event that you just have either. You can add a wide range of treats to this formula. What about some coconut, blended nuts (with the exception of peanuts), seeds, a modest quantity of cut natural product, or whatever else you want. In the event that you are stressed over calories, exclude the spread.

Sun Candies

Another name for these may be "essential fatty corrosive confections" in light of the fact that they're crammed with the stuff.

Ingredients

2½ cups sunflower seeds, ground in little clumps in the espresso processor

1½ tablespoons almond margarine

1½ tablespoons crude nectar

½ teaspoon vanilla concentrate

Preparation

Combine 2 cups ground sunflower seeds in addition to every single outstanding fixing.

Move balls in remaining ¼ cup ground sunflower seeds to cover. Serve promptly; store in icebox.

Tahini–Almond Butter Cookies

This formula originated from one of my most determined patients, Cyndi Stuart, who has investigated her own and has thought of some magnificent plans.

Ingredients

2½ cups oat flour (I make my own by hurling oats into the nourishment processor)

½ teaspoon heating powder

½ teaspoon heating pop

¾ teaspoon ocean salt

½ cup sesame margarine (tahini)

½ cup almond margarine (no salt or sugar included)

1 teaspoon vanilla

½ cup darker rice syrup

¼ cup crude nectar

¼ cup genuine maple syrup

Preparation

Preheat broiler to 350F.

In a little bowl combine the majority of the dry fixings and put in a safe spot.

With an electric blender, mix the two margarines together until smooth.

On the off chance that they become so thick that the blender experiences difficulty traveling through them, include sifted water, 1 tablespoon at once, yet close to 4 tablespoons all out.

Include the staying wet fixings, and beat on low speed until mixed.

Include the dry fixings at the same time, and beat together until well mixed. You may need to change to a wooden spoon to complete the blending.

Drop the tablespoonful onto an oiled heating sheet. Prepare until the treats are gently dark colored yet at the same time somewhat delicate, 10–12 minutes. Cool on a wire rack and serve.

Pasta With Marinara & Vegetables

Ingredients

½ cup oats, ground in an espresso processor or blender (for a thickener)

½ cup lentils, doused medium-term and water disposed of

3 enormous carrot, cut

3 celery stalks, cut

1 enormous zucchini, cut

10 shiitake mushroom, cut

1 medium sweet potato, cubed

2 cups extra boneless, skinless chicken

Chicken with Canola oil

Ingredients

1 tablespoon new ground rosemary,

1 clove minced garlic,

1/2 cup garbanzo flour,

½ cup soy flour (overlook the oat flour over),

2 eggs rather than 3,

1 tablespoon ocean salt, and ½ cup sifted water.

Preparation

Pour player in 6-inch distance across hovers rather than 3-inch and cook comparably.

Falafel

If you've ever wanted to try homemade falafel from scratch, my tutorial is all you need! Hearty and healthy vegan patties made of ground chickpeas, garlic, and fresh herbs.

Shakshuka

Turn a few eggs into the perfect meal with this simple shakshuka recipe! Eggs poached in a perfectly-spiced vegetarian stew of tomatoes and green peppers. Perfect for breakfast, lunch, or dinner.

Baked Chicken Drumsticks

The secret to these juicy, flavor-packed baked chicken drumsticks is in the marinade! Loaded with Mediterranean flavors including lemon, garlic, oregano, and extra virgin olive oil.

Greek-Style Baked Cod with Lemon and Garlic

A handful of Mediterranean spices, plus a mixture of lemon juice, olive oil, and garlic, give it glorious flavors! Comes together in just over 20 mins.

Healthy Mediterranean Chicken Orzo

With oregano, basil, parsley, olives, and feta, this orzo is practically a hall of fame for Mediterranean cuisine's biggest stars. The fresh ingredients add flavor to the whole-wheat orzo and chicken, and if the taste alone isn't incentive enough to make it, maybe the fact that it's ready in fewer than 30 minutes will be!

Harissa Pasta

Although harissa is a spice paste from North Africa, it frequently makes an appearance in Mediterranean cooking, probably thanks to the geographic proximity of the regions. Whatever the reason, we're grateful because it makes this pasta possible.